ICS 11.040.11

SCM

世界中医药学会联合会
World Federation of Chinese Medicine Societies

SCM0023-2018

热敏灸技术操作规范

Standardized Manipulations of Heat-sensitive Moxibustion Therapy

世界中联国际组织标准
International Standard of WFCMS

2018-06-24发布实施
Issued & implemented on June 24th, 2018

中医古籍出版社
Publishing House of Ancient Chinese Medical Books

图书在版编目（CIP）数据

热敏灸技术操作规范 / 世界中医药学会联合会著
.—北京：中医古籍出版社，2019.11
ISBN 978-7-5152-1945-5
Ⅰ.①热… Ⅱ.①世… Ⅲ.①艾灸—技术操作规程
Ⅳ.① R245.81-65
中国版本图书馆 CIP 数据核字（2019）第 152223 号

热敏灸技术操作规范
世界中医药学会联合会 著

责任编辑 王晓曼 张凤霞
出版发行 中医古籍出版社
社 址 北京东直门内南小街 16 号（100700）
电 话 010-64089446（总编室）010-64002949（发行部）
网 址 www.zhongyiguji.com.cn
印 刷 北京建宏印刷有限公司
开 本 880mm×1230mm 1/16
印 张 1.25
字 数 23 千字
版 次 2019 年 11 月第 1 版 2019 年 11 月第 1 次印刷
书 号 ISBN 978-7-5152-1945-5
定 价 36.00 元

目　次

前　言

本标准主要起草单位：世界中医药学会联合会热敏灸专业委员会、江西中医药大学、江西中医药大学附属医院

本标准参与起草单位：安徽中医药大学、陕西省中医医院、广东省中医院、广东省中西医结合医院、北京大学医学部、山西中医药大学、柳州市中医院、赣南医学院第一附属医院、厦门市中医院

本标准主要起草人：陈日新、陈明人、谢丁一、康明非

本标准参与起草人及审阅专家：

中　　国（以汉语拼音为序）：

曹颖、陈彦君、程爱萍、迟振海、付勇、葛宝和、洪恩四、黄国付、黄仙保、焦琳、李巧林、李勇、吕志迈、刘中勇、邱东升、苏涛、苏同生、唐福宇、田宁、田岳凤、吴春眉、徐振华、燕平、伊鸣、张波、周美启

葡 萄 牙：Frederico Carvalho

澳大利亚：Zhou Min

意 大 利：Leonardo Giovannini

日　　本：田久和义隆

加 拿 大：王建新

比 利 时：王仲彬

荷　　兰：姚奉理

本标准的起草程序遵守了世界中医药学会联合会发布的 SCM 0001–2009《标准制定和发布工作规范》和世界中医药学会联合会秘书处发布的世界中联秘发 2011（20 号）文件《世界中联各专业委员会专业技术标准制定实施办法》。

本标准在 2018 年 6 月 24 日由世界中医药学会联合会第四届第二次理事会、常务理事会与第二次监事会会议审议通过。

引　言

热敏灸是采用艾热，针对热敏腧穴施灸，通过特定手法激发透热、扩热、传热等经气传导，从而达到气至病所，并施以个体化的饱和消敏灸量，显著提高疗效的一种新灸法。

热敏灸源于经典、基于临床、继承创新，是陈日新教授带领科研团队历经30余年的科研成果，是具有自主知识产权的创新技术，无创痛、安全，患者易于接受。

现已出版的热敏灸专著有8部，其中英文版1部，日文版3部；发表论文208篇，SCI源刊25篇。2015年“热敏灸技术的创立及推广应用”项目获中华人民共和国国家科技进步二等奖。全球20余个国家与地区，约500家医院广泛应用热敏灸技术治疗脊柱关节肌肉病症、胃肠功能性病症、男性前列腺病症、女性宫寒性病症、过敏性病症、皮肤瘙痒症、亚健康等，临床疗效显著。近年来，已对20多个国家的针灸师进行了热敏灸技术的培训。为进一步促进热敏灸的传播，规范热敏灸技术操作，确保热敏灸疗效的发挥，特制定本标准。

热敏灸技术操作规范

1 范围

本标准规定了热敏灸的术语和定义、施灸前准备、操作方法与流程、适应证、注意事项等内容。

本标准适用于热敏灸技术操作。

2 规范性引用文件

下列文件对本标准的应用是必不可少的。凡是注日期的引用文件，仅注日期的版本适用于本标准。凡是不注日期的引用文件，其最新版本（包括所有的修改版）适用于本标准。

GB/T 12346–2006《腧穴名称与定位》腧穴部位。

GB/T 21709.1–2008《中华人民共和国国家标准》针灸技术操作规范第 1 部分：艾灸。

3 术语和定义

下列术语和定义适用于本标准。

3.1

热敏灸

采用艾热，针对热敏腧穴施灸，并通过特定手法激发透热、扩热、传热等经气传导，从而达到气至病所，并施以个体化的饱和消敏灸量，显著提高疗效的一种新灸法。

3.2

热敏灸感

当悬灸某个腧穴时，被灸者会产生一种深透、远传等特殊的灸感。

注：热敏灸感包括透热、扩热、传热、非热觉、肢端热、身烘热、喜热、皮肤扩散性潮红、面红（或额出汗）、胃肠蠕动反应。艾灸该腧穴邻近部位或其他某个体表部位时，被灸者仅出现局部与表面的热感，不产生以上特殊感觉。

3.3

热敏腧穴

施灸过程中产生了热敏灸感的腧穴。

3.4

艾条

以艾绒为主要成分卷成的圆柱形长条物。

注：热敏灸使用的艾条一般规格为直径：16 ～ 35mm；艾绒纯度：3 ∶ 1 ～ 8 ∶ 1。

3.5

特定手法

回旋灸、雀啄灸、循经往返灸、温和灸、接力灸及其组合手法。

4 施灸前准备

4.1 艾条选择

根据病情需要和腧穴热敏直径的不同，选择不同直径的艾条。

4.2 部位选择

依据探感定位（灸感定位法）和辨敏施灸原则，选取施灸部位。

4.3 体位选择

体位的选择以被灸者感到舒适、充分暴露施灸部位、肌肉放松为原则。

常用体位：卧位、坐位。建议首选卧位。

4.4 环境要求

同门诊治疗室的要求，并应设有排烟或消烟装置。环境温度以 24 ～ 30℃为宜。

4.5 灸感宣教

施灸者应要求被灸者在治疗过程中注意力集中，认真体会艾灸过程中的灸感，并及时与施灸者沟通交流。

5 操作方法与流程

5.1 操作方法

5.1.1 探感定位

热敏灸以灸感定位法确定热敏腧穴的位置。艾热距离体表约 3cm，以传统腧穴定位为中心，在其上下左右范围内施以回旋灸、雀啄灸、循经灸、温和灸及其组合手法进行悬灸探查，热感强度适中而无灼痛，被灸者出现 10 类热敏灸感中的 1 类或 1 类以上，此时施灸的位置即为热敏腧穴，不拘是否在传统腧穴的标准位置上。

5.1.2 辨敏施灸

辨敏施灸是通过辨别热敏腧穴的灸感特点，从而选取最优热敏腧穴施灸。按下列顺序依次选择最优穴位：以出现非热觉的热敏腧穴为首选热敏腧穴；以出现热敏灸感指向或到达病所的热敏腧穴为首选热敏腧穴；以出现较强的热敏灸感的热敏腧穴为首选热敏腧穴。

5.1.3 量因人异

进行热敏灸时，每穴、每次的施灸时间以热敏灸感消失为度，因病、因人、因穴而异，平均施灸时间约为 40min，此为热敏腧穴的最佳个体化每次施灸时间量。

5.1.4 敏消量足

只要与疾病相关的热敏腧穴存在，就需要进行疗程施灸，直至所有与该病症相关的热敏腧穴消敏，以此为治疗该病症的充足疗程灸量。

5.2 操作流程

如图 1 所示。

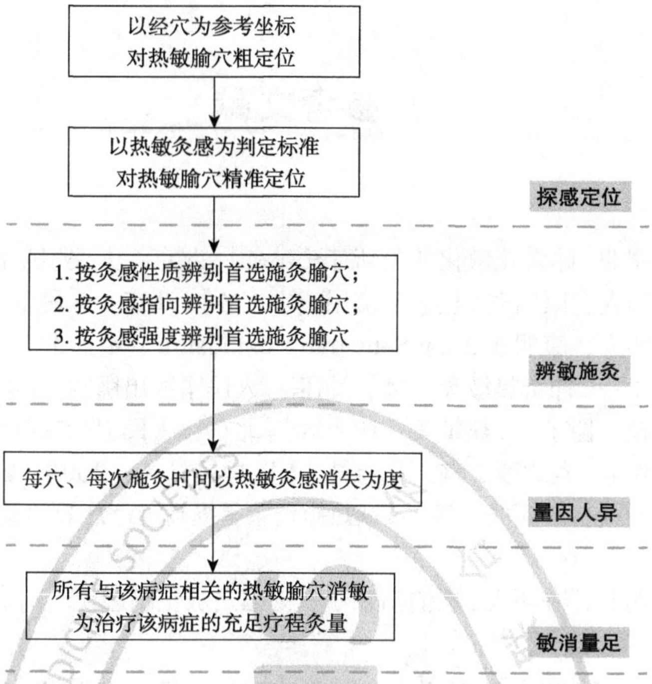

图 1　热敏灸操作流程图

6　适应证

适用于出现热敏腧穴的各种病证，不拘寒、热、虚、实、表、里等证。

7　注意事项

7.1　施灸前

施灸前，应告知被灸者艾灸过程，消除其对艾灸的恐惧感或紧张感。

7.2　施灸时

施灸时，应根据被灸者的年龄、性别、体质、病情，采取舒适的体位，并充分暴露施灸部位。操作时，应注意热感强度适宜，避免烫伤；注意防止艾火脱落，灼伤患者，或烧坏衣物。

7.3　施灸后

热敏灸结束后，须确保燃着的艾条彻底熄灭，以防复燃。施灸后，应告知被灸者在施灸结束后2h之内忌洗澡与劳累，注意保暖，避风寒。如果局部出现水疱，较小者，宜保护水疱，勿使破裂，一般数日即可吸收自愈；较大者，用注射器从水疱低位刺入，将渗出液吸出后，保持局部清洁，以防感染。

7.4　禁忌证

婴幼儿，昏迷、脑出血急性期、大量吐（咯）血的患者，过饥、过饱、过劳、酒醉等状态下的患者，孕妇的腹部和腰骶部位，感觉障碍与皮肤溃疡处不宜施灸。

参考文献

［1］陈日新，康明非．腧穴热敏化艾灸新疗法［M］．北京：人民卫生出版社，2006.

［2］陈日新，陈明人，康明非．热敏灸实用读本［M］．北京：人民卫生出版社，2009.

［3］陈日新，陈明人，康明非.Heat Sensitive Moxibusion［M］．北京：人民卫生出版社，2012.

［4］陈日新，谢丁一．神奇热敏灸［M］．北京：人民军医出版社，2013.

［5］陈日新，熊俊，谢丁一．热敏灸疗法［M］．北京：人民卫生出版社，2014.

［6］陈日新，康明非．灸之要，气至而有效［J］．中国针灸，2008，28（1）：44–46.

［7］陈日新，陈明人，康明非，等．重视热敏灸感是提高灸疗疗效的关键［J］．针刺研究，2010，35（4）：311–314.

［8］陈日新，康明非，陈明人．岐伯归来——论腧穴敏化状态说［J］．中国针灸，2011，31（2）：134–138.

［9］Xie DY，Liu ZY，Hou XQ，*et al.* Heat sensitization in suspended moxibustion：features and clinical relevance［J］. Acupunct Med，2013，31（4）：422–424.

［10］谢丁一，陈日新．悬灸得气的特征与临床应用［J］．中国针灸，2015，35（11）：1137–1139.

［11］谢丁一．陈日新教授论灸感［J］．中国针灸，2016，36（8）：789–792.

［12］陈日新，吕志迈，谢丁一，等．热敏灸得气灸感量表的研制与初步评价［J］．中国针灸，2018，38（11）：1229–1234.

［13］陈日新，吕志迈，谢丁一，等．热敏灸感条目德尔菲法调查分析［J］．中医杂志，2018，59（22）：1915–1919.

［14］谢丁一，陈日新．《内经》中腧穴二步定位法及其临床应用［J］. 中国针灸，2014，34（10）：979–982.

［15］Chen RX，Chen MR，Su TS，*et al.* Heat–sensitive moxibustion in patients with osteoarthritis of the knee：a three–armed multicenter randomized active control trial［J］. Acupunct Med，2015，33（4）：262–269.

［16］Chen MR，Chen RX，Xiong J，*et al.* Effectiveness of heat–sensitive moxibustion in the treatment of lumbar disc herniation：study protocol for a randomized controlled trial［J］. Trials，2011，12：226.

［17］Chen RX，Xiong J，Chi ZH，*et al.* Heat–sensitive moxibustion for lumbar disc herniation：a meta–analysis of randomized controlled trials［J］. Journal of Traditional Chinese Medicine，2012，32（3）：322–328.

［18］Chen RX，Chen MR，Su TS，*et al.* A 3–Arm，randomized，controlled trial of heat–sensitive moxibustion therapy to determine superior effect among patients with lumbar disc herniation［J］. Evidence–based Complementary and Alternative Medicine：eCAM，2014，2014：154941.

［19］谢丁一．热敏灸——灸疗学的传承与创新［J］．中医杂志，2016，57（11）：904–907.

［20］陈日新，谢丁一．再论"腧穴敏化状态说"［J］．安徽中医药大学学报，2016，35（3）：

50–53.

[21] Chen RX, Chen MR, Xiong J, *et al.* Is there difference between the effects of two–dose stimulation for knee osteoarthritis in the treatment of heat–sensitive Moxibustion? [J]. Evidence–based Complementary and Alternative Medicine: eCAM, 2012, 2012: 696498.

[22] Chen MR, Chen RX, Xiong J, *et al.* Evaluation of different moxibustion doses for lumbar disc herniation: multicenter randomized controlled trial of heat–sensitive moxibustion therapy [J]. Acupuncture in Medicine, 2012, 30 (4): 266–272.

Foreword

The standard is mainly drafted up by: Specialty Committee of Heat-sensitive Moxibustion of WFCMS, Jiangxi University of Traditional Chinese Medicine, Affiliated Hospital of Jiangxi University of Traditional Chinese Medicine.

Participant institutions: Anhui University of Chinese Medicine, Shaanxi Traditional Chinese Medicine Hospital, Guangdong Provincial Hospital of Chinese Medicine, Guangdong Hospital of Integrated Traditional Chinese and Western Medicine, Peking University Health Science Center, Shanxi University of Chinese Medicine, Liuzhou Traditional Chinese Medical Hospital, First Affiliated Hospital of Gannan Medical University, and Xiamen Hospital of Traditional Chinese Medicine.

The primary drafters: Chen Rixin, Chen Mingren, Xie Dingyi, and Kang Mingfei.

Drafters and review experts (Listed in alphabetical order):

China: Cao Ying, Chen Yanjun, Cheng Aiping, Chi Zhenhai, Fu Yong, Ge Baohe, Hong Ensi, Huang Guofu, Huang Xianbao, Jiao Lin, Li Qiaolin, Li Yong, Lv Zhimai, Liu Zhongyong, Qiu Dongsheng, Su Tao, Su Tongsheng, Tang Fuyu, Tian Ning, Tian Yuefeng, Wu Chunmei, Xu Zhenhua, Yan Ping, Yi Ming, Zhang Bo, Zhou Meiqi

Portugal: Frederico Carvalho

Australia: Zhou Min

Italy: Leonardo Giovannini

Japan: Takuwa Yoshitaka

Canada: Wang Jianxin

Belgium: Wang Zhongbin

Netherland: Yao Fengli

The drafting procedure of this standard complies with the WFCMS file SCM 0001-2009 <*Standard Formulated and Released Specification*> and the WFCMS file 2011 (20) <*Method for Drafting Technical Standards of WFCMS Professional Committee*>

This standard was reviewed and approved in the Second Session of the Fourth Council and Standing Council, and the Second Meeting of the Board of Supervisors of WFCMS on June 24, 2018.

Introduction

Heat-sensitive Moxibustion (HSM) is a new and effective therapy that involves moxa heat on heat-sensitive acupoints with the stimulation of specific manipulations, resulting in channel qi conduction to the affected area through heat penetration, expanding and transmission. With sufficient individual moxibustion dosage that eliminates the heat sensitization, HSM can significantly enhance the therapeutic effects.

Based on the TCM classics and clinical experience, Professor Chen Rixin and his research team studied for over 30 years and invented HSM, which is an original innovative technology with independent intellectual property rights. As a noninvasive, painless and safe therapy, HSM is easily accepted by patients.

Up to now, 8 HSM monographs have been published, including one English version, three Japanese versions, and 208 papers have been published, with 25 in SCI Source Journals. In 2015, the project of "The creation and popularizing application of HSM" won the Second Class Prize of the State Scientific and Technological Progress Award of China. HSM has been put into use in more than 500 hospitals in over 20 countries and regions for treating spinal, joint and muscle diseases, functional gastrointestinal disorders, prostate diseases, disorders due to uterus cold, allergic disorders, cutaneous itching, and improving sub-health status, etc, greatly improving the clinical efficacy. In recent years, acupuncturists from more than 20 countries have been trained with the HSM technique. There is a desperate need for HSM standard in order to promote HSM'S international communication, standardize its manipulations, and ensure its efficacy, thus, this standard is made.

Standardized Manipulation of Heat-Sensitive Moxibustion Therapy

1 Scope

This standard specifies the terms and definitions, preparations before moxibustion, operation methods and procedure, indications and cautions of HSM therapy.

This standard is applicable to the HSM therapy.

2 Normative references

The following referenced documents are indispensable for the application of this standard. For dated references, only the edition cited applies. For undated references, the latest edition of the referenced document (including any amendments) applies.

GB/T 12346–2006 *Name and Location of Acupoint*, (the part of acupoint)

GB/T 21709.1–2008 *The State Standard of the People's Republic of China, Standardized Manipulations of Acupuncture and Moxibustion*, (Chapter 1: Moxibustion)

3 Terms and definitions

For the purposes of this document, the following terms and definitions are applied.

3.1

Heat-sensitive moxibustion therapy (HSM)

It is a new and effective therapy that involves moxa heat on heat-sensitive acupoints with the stimulation of specific manipulations, resulting in channel qi conduction to the affected area through heat penetration, expanding and transmission, *etc*. With sufficient individual moxibustion dosage, HSM can significantly enhance the therapeutic effect.

3.2

Sensations due to HSM

When administered suspended moxibustion on the body surface of certain enhance, the patient will have special sensations like heat penetration or transmission.

Note: Sensations due to HSM include heat penetration, heat expanding, heat transmission, non-heat sensation, acra-heat, whole body warm, a preferring to warm, diffusible flushing on the skin, facial flushing (or sweating on the forehead), and gastrointestinal peristalsis. When applying moxibustion on the point near the acupoint or other part on the body surface, the patient only feel warm in local or superficial part without the above mentioned special feelings.

3.3

Heat-sensitive acupoints

The points on which the HSM sensations can be elicited by moxibustion.

3.4

Moxa stick

A cylindrical stick mainly made with moxa being rolled

Note: General specification of moxa stick used in HSM: 16 ~35 mm in diameter; moxa purity: 3:1-8:1.

3.5

Specific manipulations

Circling moxibustion, sparrow-pecking moxibustion, back-and-forth moxibustion along channels, mild moxibustion, relay moxibustion and combination of five manipulations above mentioned.

4 Preparations before moxibustion

4.1 Moxa stick selection

Moxa stick with different diameter is selected according to the disease condition and the range of acupoint heat-sensitization.

4.2 Area selection

The area for HSM is selected based on the method of locating acupoint by sensation due to HSM and principle of selecting optimal heat-sensitive acupoint.

4.3 Body posture selection

The body posture is selected based on the principles of comfortable feeling of those who accept HSM, full exposure of the therapeutic area and muscle relaxation.

Common body postures: recumbent, prone and sitting positions. The former two are recommended.

4.4 Environmental requirements

It is the same to the outpatient treatment room. Besides, there should be a fume extractor or smoke eliminating equipment. The temperature should be kept in 24-30 ℃ .

4.5 HSM sensations acknowledgement

The performers should ask those who accept HSM to focus on the sensations during moxibustion, and to communicate with them promptly.

5 Operation methods and procedure

5.1 Operation methods

5.1.1 Locating acupoint by sensation

HSM locates the heat-sensitive acupoints according to the sensations due to HSM. Keeping 3 centimeters between the burning moxa stick and body surface, the exploration of heat-sensitive acupoints is performed around the traditional acupoint location by circling moxibustion, sparrow-pecking moxibustion, back-and forth moxibustion along channels, mild moxibustion and combination of the manipulations mentioned above. And the moxibustion heat should be moderate without burning pain. If those who accept moxibustion feel one or more types of HSM sensations when moxibustion on a certain point, it is where the heat-sensitive acupoint locates, regardless of the traditional standard position of acupoint.

5.1.2 Selecting optimal heat-sensitive acupoint

The HSM sensations may appear in several acupoints. Thus according to the characteristics of sensation of each acupoints, the optimal heat-sensitive acupoint is selected in the following order of priority: acupoints that exhibit non-heat sensations; the acupoints where HSM sensations appear and trend to the area of diseases; acupoints where a strong HSM sensation appears.

5.1.3 Varying the dosage individually

Moxibustion each time on each acupoint is finished when HSM sensation disappears, it varies from disease to disease, from person to person, and from acupoint to acupoint. The average time is about 40 minutes, which is the optimal individual HSM time.

5.1.4 Ending after sufficient dosage

As long as heat-sensitive acupoints associated diseases exist, there is a need for moxibustion. When the sensitization of all acupoints relevant to the disease disappears, the whole therapy comes to the end. It is regarded as the sufficient effective dosage of HSM therapy.

5.2 Operation procedure (Fig. 1)

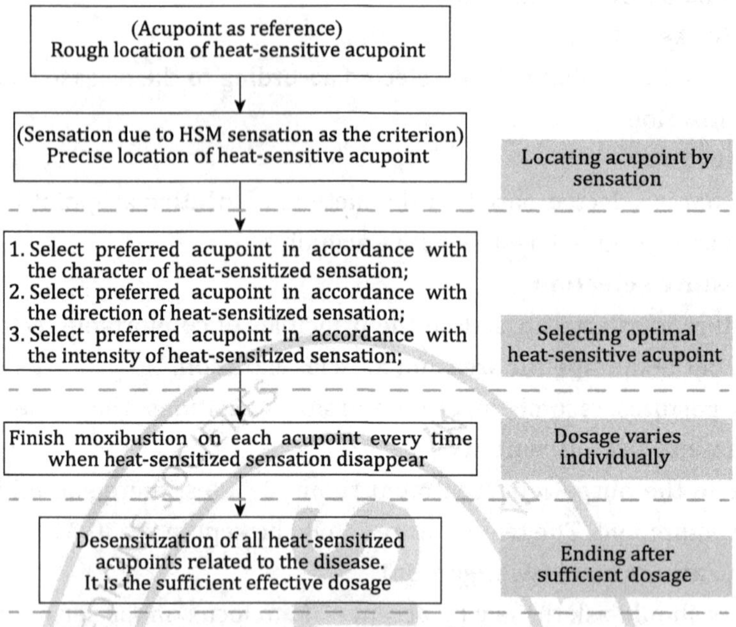

Fig. 1 Operation procedure of HSM therapy

6 Indications

It is suitable for various diseases and syndromes where heat-sensitive acupoints can be found, irrespective of cold, heat, deficiency, excess, exterior or interior syndromes.

7 Cautions

7.1 Before therapy

Those who accept moxibustion should be explained about the whole process in order to eliminate their fear or tension.

7.2 During therapy

A comfortable body posture is taken according to the age, gender, body constitution and disease condition, and the area for moxibustion should be fully exposed. During the therapy, the moxibustion temperature and intensity should be appropriate burns. In addition, the burning stick should be prevented from falling off and burning patients, clothes or other things.

7.3 After therapy

After the therapy, the burning moxa stick must be extinguished completely to prevent reburn. Those who accept moxibustion should be informed that they should not take a shower in two hours after therapy and should avoid win-cold and keep warm. As to blisters in local area, if the blister is small, it should be protected from broken, which usually absorbed and healed by itself a few days later; if the blister is big, it should be punctured at the bottom with a syringe. After the exudation is extracted out, keep the local area clean to prevent infection.

7.4 Contraindications

Infants, patients with coma, acute phase of cerebral hemorrhage, or hematemesis (hemoptysis) in large amounts, or in the condition such as hunger, satiety, overwork and drunk; abdomen and lumbosacral region of a pregnant woman; local area with sensory disorder or skin ulcer.

Bibliography

[1] Chen RX, Kang MF: Heat-Sensitization of Acupoint, a New Moxibustion Therapy [M] . Beijing: People's Medical Publishing House, 2006.

[2] Chen RX, Chen MR, Kang MF: Practical Reading of Heat-Sensitization Moxibustion [M] . Beijing: People's Medical Publishing House, 2009.

[3] Chen RX, Chen MR, Kang MF: Heat Sensitive Moxibustion [M] . Beijing: People's Medical Publishing House, 2009.

[4] Chen RX, Xie DY: Magic Heat-sensitive Moxibustion [M] . Beijing: People's Military Medical Publisher, 2013.

[5] Chen RX, Xiong J, Xie DY: Heat-Sensitive Moxibustion Therapy [M] . Beijing: People's Medical Publishing House, 2014.

[6] Chen RX, Kang MF. Key Point of Moxibustion, Arrival of Qi produces curative effect [J] . Chinese Acupuncture & Moxibustion, 2008, 28(1): 44-46.

[7] Chen RX, Chen MR, Kang MF *et al.* Paying attention to the heat thermal sensitivity of Moxibustion Is The Key for Raising the Curative Effect [J] . Acupuncture Research, 2010, 35(4) : 311-314.

[8] Chen RX, Kang MF, Chen MR. Return of Qibo: on hypothesis of sensitization state of acupoints [J]. Chinese Acupuncture & Moxibustion, 2011, 31(2): 134-138.

[9] Xie DY, Liu ZY, Hou XQ, *et al.* Heat sensitization in suspended moxibustion: features and clinical relevance [J] . Acupunct Med, 2013, 31(4): 422-424.

[10] Xie DY, Chen RX. Characteristics and Clinical Application of the Arrival of Qi in Suspended Moxibustion [J] . Chinese Acupuncture & Moxibustion, 2015, 35(11): 1137-1139.

[11] Xie DY. Professor Chen Rixin's view on moxibustion sensation [J] .Chinese Acupuncture & Moxibustion, 2016, 36(8): 789-792.

[12] Chen RX, Lv ZM, Xie DY *et al.* Development andinitial evaluation of Deqi sensation scale of heat-sensitive moxibustion [J] . Chinese Acupuncture & Moxibustion, 2018, 38(11), 1229-1234.

[13] Chen RX, Lv ZM, Xie DY, *et al.* Investigation and analysis of heat-sensitive moxibustion sensation items by delphi method [J] . Journal of Traditional Chinese Medicine, 2018, 59(22), 1915-1919

[14] Xie DY, Chen RX. The two-step location method of acupoint in *Internal Canon of Medicine* and its clinical application [J] . Chinese Acupuncture & Moxibustion, 2014, 34(10): 979-982.

[15] Chen RX, Chen MR, Su TS, *et al.* Heat-sensitive moxibustion in patients with osteoarthritis of the knee: a three-armed multicenter randomized active control trial [J] . Acupunct Med, 2015, 33(4): 262-269.

[16] Chen MR, Chen RX, Xiong J, *et al.* Effectiveness of heat-sensitive moxibustion in the treatment of lumbar disc herniation: study protocol for a randomized controlled trial [J] . Trials, 2011, 12: 226.

[17] Chen RX, Xiong J, Chi ZH, *et al.* Heat-sensitive moxibustion for lumbar disc herniation: a meta-analysis of randomized controlled trials[J] . Journal of Traditional Chinese Medicine, 2012, 32(3): 322-328.

[18] Chen RX, Chen MR, Su TS, *et al.* A 3-Arm, randomized, controlled trial of heat-sensitive moxibustion therapy to determine superior effect among patients with lumbar disc herniation [J] . Evidence-based Complementary and Alternative Medicine: eCAM, 2014, 2014: 154941.

[19] Xie DY. Heat-sensitive moxibustion: inheritance and innovation of moxibustion theory [J] . Journal of Traditional Chinese Medicine, 2016, 57(11): 904-907.

[20] Chen RX, Xie DY. Further Discussion on "the hypothesis of sensitization state of acupoints" [J]. Journal of Anhui Traditional Chinese Medicine College, 2016, 35(3): 50-53.

[21] Chen RX, Chen MR, Xiong J, *et al.* Is there difference between the effects of two-dose stimulation for knee osteoarthritis in the treatment of heat-sensitive Moxibustion? [J] . Evidence-based Complementary and Alternative Medicine: eCAM, 2012, 2012: 696498.

[22] Chen MR, Chen RX, Xiong J, *et al.* Evaluation of different moxibustion doses for lumbar disc herniation: multicenter randomized controlled trial of heat-sensitive moxibustion therapy [J] . Acupuncture in Medicine, 2012, 30(4): 266-272.